MACULAR DEGENERATION MANAGEMENT DIET COOKBOOK

Optimal Vision Recipes: Nourish Your Sight Naturally–Nutrition Solutions For Clearer Eyesight –Eat Your Way To Brighter Vision

DR. SHAYLA LEWIS

Table of Contents

DISCLAIMER

Write a brief complete Disclaimer for my diet cook book telling them that the author is not in any association with any company, business or individual and also this book is written by the authors knowledge and understanding

The information provided in this diet cookbook is based on the author's personal knowledge and understanding. The author is not affiliated with, endorsed by, or associated with any company, business, or individual. The recipes and dietary advice contained within this book are intended for informational purposes only. Readers should consult with a healthcare professional or a registered dietitian before making any significant changes to their diet or lifestyle. The author assumes no responsibility for any adverse effects that may result from the use or misuse of the information contained in this book.

CHAPTER ONE

The Fundamentals of Macular Degeneration Treatment Diet

Glaucoma Prevention Diet Cookbook delves deeply into the dietary methods required to manage macular degeneration, a common eye condition that affects millions of people around the world. This chapter looks into the underlying ideas required to understand macular degeneration and how nutrition plays a critical role in its treatment.

Explaining Macular Degeneration and its Types: Macular degeneration, also known as age-related macular degeneration (AMD), is a degenerative eye illness that predominantly affects the macula, the center region of the retina that provides sharp, central vision. AMD can be classified into two types: "dry" (atrophic) and "wet" (exudative or neovascular). Dry AMD is defined by the slow loss of light-sensitive cells in the macula, whereas wet AMD is characterized by aberrant blood vessel growth beneath the eye, which causes leaking and damage.

Overview of Nutrition's Role in Treating the Condition: Nutrition is critical in treating macular degeneration, with evidence indicating that specific foods can help slow its progression and lessen the likelihood of acquiring advanced stages of the illness. Antioxidants including vitamins C and E, zinc, lutein, zeaxanthin, and omega-3 fatty acids are essential nutrients.

These nutrients help protect the retina from oxidative damage, inflammation, and aberrant blood vessel creation, which preserves vision and slows disease progression.

Understanding the Importance of Low-Carb, Antioxidant-Rich, and Anti-Inflammatory

Foods: A macular degeneration management diet focuses on low-carb, antioxidant-rich foods with anti-inflammatory qualities. Low-carb diets help to regulate blood sugar levels, which is essential for maintaining overall eye health. Antioxidant-rich foods like fruits, vegetables, nuts, and seeds assist to neutralise free radicals and reduce oxidative stress in the retina. Anti-inflammatory foods, such as fatty fish, olive oil, turmeric, and leafy greens, also aid in reducing eye inflammation and maintain good ocular health.

Tips for Creating a Balanced Diet Plan:

To manage macular degeneration, incorporate a range of nutrient-dense meals that contain vital vitamins, minerals, antioxidants, and omega-3 fatty acids. A nutritious diet should consist of a variety of colorful fruits and vegetables, lean proteins, whole grains, healthy fats, and low-fat dairy products. It's also crucial to restrict your consumption of processed meals, sugary snacks, and unhealthy fats, which can all contribute to inflammation and oxidative stress in the body.

Grocery Shopping Guide: Choosing the correct products: Navigating the grocery store can be intimidating, but using a shopping guide will help you choose the correct products for a macular degeneration management diet. Look for fresh food, such as leafy greens, berries, carrots, and bell peppers, which are high in antioxidants and critical nutrients for vision. Choose lean protein sources such as poultry, fish, tofu, and lentils, as well as nutritious grains like quinoa, brown rice, and oats. Make sure to stock up on healthy fats like olive oil, almonds, and seeds, as well as low-fat dairy products and omega-3-rich meals like salmon and flaxseeds. By making wise grocery store purchases, you may prepare delicious and healthy meals that promote eye health and general well-being.

Essential Nutrients for Macular Degeneration Management.

Vitamin A: The Essential Nutrient for Eye Health.

Vitamin A is essential for keeping clear vision, especially in low-light circumstances. It is an essential component of rhodopsin, a protein in the retina that aids in night vision. Additionally, vitamin A promotes the health of the cornea and other eye tissues. A lack of vitamin A can cause night blindness, which makes it difficult to see in low light. Incorporating vitamin A-rich foods into your diet, such as carrots, sweet potatoes, spinach, kale, and liver, can help maintain good eye health and prevent visual difficulties caused by vitamin A deficiency.

The Importance of Omega-3 Fatty Acids in preventing progression

Omega-3 fatty acids are necessary lipids that the body cannot manufacture and must be received from diet.

These fats are recognized for their anti-inflammatory characteristics, which can help reduce eye irritation and protect against diseases such as macular degeneration. Omega-3 fatty acids, notably EPA (eicosapentaenoic acid) and DHA (docosahexaenoic acid), have been shown in studies to reduce the course of macular degeneration and preserve vision. Omega-3 fatty acids are found in fatty fish such as salmon, mackerel, and sardines, as well as flaxseeds, chia seeds, and walnuts.

Antioxidants protect against free radical damage.

Antioxidants are substances that help neutralize free radicals, which are unstable molecules that can harm cells, including those in the eyes. Antioxidants help defend against oxidative stress and inflammation, both of which have been linked to the development and progression of macular degeneration. Vitamin C, vitamin E, lutein, zeaxanthin, and beta-carotene are among the most important antioxidants for eye health. Citrus fruits, almonds, leafy greens, and bell peppers are examples of foods rich in antioxidants.

Minerals and Their Impact on Eye Health
Several minerals are vital for preserving eye health and preventing disorders such as macular degeneration. Zinc, for example, has a role in vitamin A metabolism and

contributes to retinal structure. Zinc supplementation has been found in studies to decrease the course of macular degeneration in some patients. Other minerals, such as selenium and copper, also help with overall eye health. Foods high in these minerals include oysters, meat, chicken, nuts, seeds, and whole grains.

Incorporating Fibre for Overall Health

While fiber is not as directly linked to eye health as vitamins and minerals, it is important for general wellness, which can have an indirect impact on eye health. A fiber-rich diet helps maintain healthy blood sugar levels and promotes cardiovascular health, both of which are essential for optimal eye performance. Additionally, fiber-rich foods such as fruits, vegetables, whole grains, and legumes are high in vitamins, minerals, and antioxidants, which promote overall eye health. By including fiber-rich foods in your diet, you can enhance your overall health and lower your risk of acquiring illnesses such as macular degeneration.

CHAPTER TWO

Developing Low-Carb, Antioxidant-Rich, and Anti-Inflammatory Meals

The Glaucoma Prevention Diet Cookbook emphasizes the necessity of creating meals that are both enjoyable and precisely designed to benefit eye health. In this chapter, we will look at the principles of low-carb, antioxidant-rich, and anti-inflammatory diets, which have an important role in reducing the risk factors for glaucoma.

Low-carbohydrate meals:

Low-carb meals are vital for controlling blood sugar levels, which improves overall health, including eye health. Excess carbohydrate intake can cause insulin resistance and inflammation, both of which are harmful to eye health. Individuals who choose low-carb diets can control their blood sugar levels and lower their chance of acquiring glaucoma.

The cookbook contains a variety of low-carb meal options, including breakfast meals, snacks, and desserts. These meals are intended to be both enjoyable and nutrient-dense, allowing people to maintain a healthy diet while sticking to their specific dietary choices and needs.

Antioxidant-Rich Foods:
Antioxidants are essential for protecting the eyes from oxidative stress, which contributes significantly to the development and progression of glaucoma. Individuals who incorporate antioxidant-rich foods into their diet can improve their eye health and minimize their risk of glaucoma-related vision loss.

Our cookbook has a variety of antioxidant-rich recipes, including those high in fruits, vegetables, nuts, and seeds. These nutrients are rich in vitamins, minerals, and phytochemicals, which not only benefit eye health but also contribute to general well-being.

Chronic inflammation is linked to a variety of ocular diseases, including glaucoma. Individuals who follow an anti-inflammatory diet can lower inflammation and the chance of getting glaucoma or experiencing its side effects.

We provide a variety of anti-inflammatory meals with elements known for their anti-inflammatory qualities. These contain omega-3 fatty acids, turmeric, ginger, leafy greens, and good fats. Individuals who prioritize these foods can help reduce inflammation and improve their eyes' long-term health.

Simple and nutritious breakfast ideas:

Breakfast is widely regarded as the most essential meal of the day and with good reason. A good meal can set the tone for the rest of the day, giving people the energy and nutrients they require to thrive.

In this part, we share simple but substantial breakfast recipes that are quick to make and high in key nutrients. Our breakfast recipes cater to a wide range of tastes and nutritional preferences, including smoothie bowls, chia pudding, egg muffins, and avocado toast.

Wholesome Lunch Options for Sustained Energy:

Lunchtime provides an opportunity to replenish and rejuvenate, guaranteeing consistent energy throughout the day. Our cookbook has a variety of healthy lunch options that are intended to keep people feeling pleased and energized until their next meal.

Our lunch options, which range from substantial salads and grain bowls to wraps and soups, have a balanced amount of protein, fiber, and healthy fats to encourage satiety and general health. These meals are easy to prepare and may be tailored to individual preferences and dietary requirements.

Delicious Dinner Recipes that Promote Healing:

Dinner is a time to relax and replenish the body after a long day. Our cookbook features a variety of delectable dinner dishes that not only satisfy but also encourage healing and well-being.

Our dinner recipes prioritize flavor and nutrition, with everything from warming stews and stir-fries to oven-roasted vegetables and protein-packed main dishes. These meals provide a balanced macronutrient and micronutrient profile by using a range of healthful items.

Snacks and sweets do not have to be decadent to be pleasurable. Our cookbook includes a variety of delicious and nutritious snacks and desserts, allowing people to satisfy their desires without jeopardizing their health goals.

Our dishes range from energy balls and fruit skewers to yogurt parfaits and dark chocolate delights, providing healthier alternatives to typical snacks and desserts. These delights, which use healthful ingredients and limit added sugars and refined carbohydrates, give a guilt-free way to indulge while promoting eye health.

Hydration: Importance and Creative Drink Options:

Hydration is critical to general health, including eye health. Adequate hydration promotes fluid homeostasis in the body and supports a variety of physiological activities, including circulation and detoxification.

This section emphasizes the significance of being hydrated and offers inventive beverage options to assist people achieve their daily fluid demands. Our recipes range from infused waters and herbal teas to smoothies and homemade electrolyte drinks, providing a delicious way to stay hydrated while also supporting eye health.

Individuals who include these principles and recipes in their everyday routines can take proactive actions to prevent glaucoma and promote their eyes' long-term health. With a focus on low-carb, antioxidant-rich, and anti-inflammatory meals, our cookbook enables people to make informed dietary decisions that prioritize their eye health and general well-being.

CHAPTER THREE

Meal Planning and Preparation Made Easy

Meal planning and preparation are critical components of maintaining a balanced diet, especially for illnesses such as glaucoma. This chapter discusses how to make meal planning and preparation more practical, efficient, and pleasant for people who want to add glaucoma-friendly foods to their diet.

Weekly Meal Plan Strategies:

Weekly meal planning entails choosing recipes and arranging meals for the coming week. Individuals with glaucoma should consume foods rich in nutrients such as vitamins A, C, and E, as well as omega-3 fatty acids while minimizing sodium intake. Creating a weekly meal plan ensures balanced nutrition and decreases the temptation to eat less healthful foods.

Consider adding a variety of fruits, vegetables, whole grains, lean meats, and healthy fats to your meals. Experiment with new recipes and flavors to make meals more interesting and pleasurable. Use internet tools, cookbooks, and apps to explore new recipes for glaucoma prevention.

Batch cooking is the process of making big amounts of food ahead of time and storing parts for later use. This technique can save time and effort on hectic weekdays while still providing access to healthful meals. When batch cooking for glaucoma prevention, use recipes that contain components known for their eye health advantages.

Choose meals that include leafy greens, colorful fruits and vegetables, nuts, seeds, and omega-3-rich fish. Soups, stews, casseroles, and grain-based salads are ideal for batch cooking. Invest in high-quality storage containers to keep batch-cooked foods fresh in the fridge or freezer.

Proper storage practices are essential for preserving the freshness and quality of food, especially when cooking meals ahead. To avoid deterioration and extend shelf life, store perishable foods such as fruits, vegetables, and cooked proteins in airtight containers. Consider investing in specialized storage containers that will keep producing fresher for longer periods.

Keep fruits and vegetables separate to avoid early ripening and rotting.

To keep leafy greens and herbs crisp, store them on damp paper towels. Label containers with the date of preparation to maintain freshness and guarantee timely consumption. Additionally, clear out the refrigerator and pantry regularly to get rid of expired products and reduce food wastage.

Quick and easy meal prep ideas are vital for busy people who want to eat healthy without losing time or convenience. When planning meals for glaucoma prevention, choose foods that are easy, nutritional, and enjoyable. Choose meals with low preparation time and excellent nutritional value.

For a quick and healthy breakfast, try overnight oats or chia seed pudding. Create colorful salads with leafy greens, chopped vegetables, and protein sources such as grilled chicken or tofu. Invest in pre-cut vegetables and pre-cooked grains to simplify meal preparation and save time in the kitchen.

Tools and Appliances for Effective Cooking:

Efficient cooking requires the proper tools and appliances to speed meal preparation. Invest in kitchen tools such as sharp knives, cutting boards, measuring cups, and mixing bowls to make cooking easier. Consider acquiring a food processor or blender to help you swiftly chop vegetables, make sauces, and blend smoothies.

Slow cookers and instant pots are also useful gadgets for hands-free cooking and menu variety. These gadgets are ideal for making soups, stews, and one-pot meals with little effort. A high-quality nonstick skillet or grill pan can also make cooking easier and reduce the need for additional fats or oils.

In conclusion, meal planning and preparation are critical components of maintaining a glaucoma-prevention diet. Individuals can simplify the process of adding nutritious foods to their diet by using weekly meal planning tactics, batch cooking advice, proper storage procedures, quick and easy meal prep ideas, and the right tools and appliances.

Navigating Menus for Healthy Options: Dining out may be both enjoyable and challenging, especially if you're attempting to stick to a glaucoma-prevention diet. However, with some clever tactics, you can still eat in restaurants while making healthy selections. When browsing the menu, search for foods high in nutrients such as vitamins A, C, and E, as well as antioxidants and omega-3 fatty acids, which are good for your eyes. To cut down on bad fats, choose grilled, roasted, or steamed foods over fried ones.

Many restaurants now provide lighter meals or "health-conscious" sections on their menus, making it easier to select appropriate options. Please do not hesitate to ask your server for recommendations or dietary changes. For example, you can request that foods be prepared with less salt and oil, or that vegetables be given as a side dish instead of fries.

Tips for Making Smart Restaurant Choices: When dining out, it's critical to pay attention to portion sizes and avoid indulging in high-calorie, high-sodium items. Consider sharing entrees with your dinner friends or ordering appetizers or starters as your main course. Choose lean proteins such as fish, poultry, or tofu, along with lots of veggies and healthful grains.

Condiments and sauces should be used with caution because they can include hidden sugars and harmful fat. Ask for dressings and sauces on the side so you may control how much you eat. Additionally, be cautious of alcoholic beverages, since excessive consumption can raise intraocular pressure and worsen glaucoma symptoms. Choose water, herbal tea, or fresh fruit juice as healthier options.

How to Handle Social Gatherings and Events: Adhering to a glaucoma-prevention diet can be difficult at times. However, with some thought and preparation, you can easily manage these circumstances.

Before attending an event, ask about the menu or meal alternatives.

If possible, offer to bring food that is compatible with your dietary choices and constraints, ensuring that you have at least one healthy option.

At gatherings, prioritize socializing and enjoying the company of others over the food. Practice mindful eating by savoring each bite and paying attention to hunger and fullness signals. If you are presented with tempting snacks or unhealthy selections, allow yourself to indulge in moderation while balancing it with better choices throughout the day.

Communicating Your Dietary Needs Effectively: Effective communication is essential for ensuring that your dietary needs are addressed, particularly in social settings. Be proactive in advising hosts or restaurant personnel about your dietary limitations and preferences, emphasizing the significance of sticking to your glaucoma-prevention diet. If necessary, make recommendations or alternatives, and thank everybody who made an effort to accommodate you.

If you run into any challenges or misconceptions, be nice and patient while clarifying your needs. Remember that most people are willing to accommodate dietary limitations, especially if they recognize the value of being healthy.

Bringing Your Own Dish: Potluck and Party Ideas: Bringing your own dish to a potluck or party guarantees that you have something nutritious to eat while also allowing you to share your favorite recipes with others.

When selecting a dish to offer, choose nutrient-dense options such as salads, vegetable-based dishes, or whole-grain casseroles. Consider using nutrients known to improve eye health, such as leafy greens, colorful vegetables, and nuts.

If you're confused about what to make, there are numerous glaucoma-friendly recipes available online or in specialized cookbooks. Choose meals that are portable and can be served at room temperature, avoiding the need for reheating or refrigeration. Label your food with a list of ingredients to assist visitors with dietary restrictions or allergies in identifying suitable options.

Overall, with careful planning and a little imagination, dining out and socializing may be fun while following a glaucoma-prevention diet. You may maintain ideal eye health without jeopardizing your social life by making wise decisions, communicating effectively, and being proactive about your nutritional needs.

CHAPTER FOUR

Treating Macular Degeneration
Symptoms Naturally

Understanding Common Symptoms and Triggers:

Macular degeneration is a disorder that affects the macula, a small but important part of the retina responsible for central vision. As the condition advances, people may notice blurred or distorted vision, black or empty regions in the center of their vision, and difficulties seeing colors clearly. Understanding these symptoms and their triggers is critical for successful therapy.

Age, heredity, smoking, a poor diet, and exposure to harmful UV rays are common triggers for macular degeneration symptoms, however, they might vary by individual. Recognizing these triggers allows individuals to make proactive efforts to reduce their influence and maybe prevent the advancement of the disease.

Lifestyle Changes for Eye Health:

A healthy lifestyle can considerably improve eye health and even alleviate the symptoms of macular degeneration. This involves making dietary changes, quitting smoking, controlling weight, and shielding the eyes from dangerous UV radiation. A Glaucoma Prevention Diet Cookbook can help you incorporate nutrient-rich meals that enhance eye health while avoiding harmful ingredients.

Stress Management Strategies for Overall Wellness:

Stress can increase macular degeneration symptoms while also hurting overall health. Stress management approaches such as meditation, deep breathing exercises, yoga, and mindfulness can be quite effective. These strategies assist patients in developing a sense of calm, reducing worry, and promoting overall well-being, which can indirectly lead to better management of macular degeneration symptoms.

Regular exercise is important for treating macular degeneration symptoms and improving overall health. Physical activity increases blood circulation, which is necessary for delivering oxygen and nutrients to the eyes. Exercise also helps to maintain a healthy weight, decreases inflammation, and promotes optimal cardiovascular function, all of which contribute to improved eye health and symptom management.

Integrating Relaxation and Mindfulness Practices:

Relaxation and mindfulness methods can help people manage macular degeneration symptoms. Progressive muscle relaxation, guided imagery, and mindfulness meditation are all techniques that can aid with stress reduction, mood improvement, and general well-being. Individuals who include these practices in their daily lives can build resilience, manage more successfully with obstacles, and feel better clarity and peace of mind despite the uncertainties of living with macular degeneration.

By incorporating these ideas into a Glaucoma Prevention Diet Cookbook, people can gain access to a comprehensive resource that not only provides nutritious recipes but also equips them with knowledge and strategies for naturally managing macular degeneration symptoms and improving their overall quality of life.

The Glaucoma Prevention Diet Cookbook recognizes that going on a dietary journey to prevent or manage glaucoma can bring its own set of challenges. This chapter goes deeply into resolving these concerns, offering practical insights and answers to promote a seamless and successful transition to a healthier lifestyle.

Potential Side Effects of Dietary Changes

Transitioning to a new diet can have unforeseen negative effects. Individuals may feel temporary discomfort or alterations in physical processes as a result of abrupt changes in nutritional consumption or when the body adjusts to new diets. The Glaucoma Prevention Diet Cookbook addresses these potential adverse effects and advises on how to successfully manage them. From digestive difficulties to changes in energy levels, readers are given advice on how to deal with these challenges while remaining dedicated to their eating goals.

Dealing with food allergies and sensitivities Food allergies and sensitivities might make it difficult to switch to a new diet. The cookbook emphasizes the significance of identifying and managing any potential allergens or sensitivities to achieve the best health outcomes. Readers are shown how to read food labels, substitute ingredients, and locate appropriate alternatives without sacrificing nutritional quality or flavor. By offering a variety of customizable recipes and ingredient combinations, the cookbook allows people to adjust their diet to their own nutritional needs and interests.

Eating healthily does not have to be prohibitively expensive. In this part, the Glaucoma Prevention Diet Cookbook looks at low-cost ways to incorporate nutrient-dense foods into your everyday meals. From low-cost protein sources to cost-effective methods to incorporate fresh fruits and vegetables, readers will be prepared with practical techniques for maximizing nutritious value while staying within their budget. The cookbook shows that eating properly can be both accessible and economical for everyone by emphasizing the significance of meal planning, smart purchasing, and using cost-effective foods.

CHAPTER FIVE

Plateaus are common on any wellness journey, including dietary adjustments intended to avoid glaucoma. Whether it's a weight loss plateau or a stall in health improvements, the cookbook offers techniques for overcoming these roadblocks and resuming progress. Readers are advised to be patient and persistent in their pursuit of better health outcomes, whether it is by modifying portion sizes or introducing diversity into meals. The cookbook enables people to break through plateaus and keep advancing toward their health objectives by emphasizing the significance of consistency and making small changes over time.

Seeking support from family, friends, and support groups.

Starting a diet can be intimidating, but it doesn't have to be done alone. The Glaucoma Prevention Diet Cookbook emphasizes the need to request help from loved ones and community resources.

Readers are advised to surround themselves with a supportive network, whether that means enlisting the help of family members in meal preparation or joining a support group for others with similar health goals.

The cookbook promotes a sense of community and accountability, which helps people stay motivated and dedicated to their nutritional goals. It also offers advice on how to properly explain nutritional preferences to friends and family members, resulting in a helpful and understanding atmosphere for everyone.

In this chapter of the Glaucoma Prevention Diet Cookbook, we will look at some of the most often-asked questions about the role of diet in managing macular degeneration. It is natural to have questions and concerns as you begin your path toward better eye health. Let us investigate these questions in depth to provide you with the clarity and assistance you require.

Can Diet Really Help with Macular Degeneration?

The short answer is yes, nutrition can help manage macular degeneration. While genetics and other factors undoubtedly contribute to the formation and advancement of this disorder, research suggests that some nutrients can promote eye health and potentially decrease the onset of macular degeneration.

Foods high in antioxidants, vitamins, and minerals, including lutein, zeaxanthin, vitamin C, vitamin E, zinc, and omega-3 fatty acids, have been demonstrated to improve eye health. These nutrients serve to protect the eyes from oxidative stress, inflammation, and free radical damage. By including a range of nutrient-dense foods in your diet, you may provide your eyes with the nutrients they require to stay healthy and perform properly.

How Soon Can I See Results From Dietary Changes?

The timing for noticing outcomes from dietary changes varies from person to person. While some people notice improvements in their eye health right away, others may see more gradual changes over time. It is vital to realize that dietary adjustments may not be sufficient to reverse or totally stop macular degeneration. However, a balanced diet can supplement other treatment options and improve general eye health.

Consistency is essential for seeing outcomes from dietary modifications. It may take several weeks or even months of faithfully following a macular degeneration-friendly diet to see improvements in your symptoms or general eye health. Be patient and commit to making good choices every day.

Which foods should I avoid to avoid symptom flare-ups?

While some foods can benefit eye health, others may aggravate symptoms or contribute to inflammation and oxidative stress in the eyes. Some foods to limit or avoid include processed foods high in refined carbohydrates and harmful fats, as well as sodium-rich foods.

Furthermore, people with macular degeneration may be susceptible to specific dietary ingredients including saturated fats and cholesterol. It is critical to consult with a healthcare practitioner or certified dietitian to decide which foods are best for you and your individual nutritional requirements.

Can supplements improve the effects of a Macular Degeneration Diet?

In some circumstances, supplements may be prescribed to augment a macular degeneration diet and ensure optimal vitamin intake. Omega-3 fatty acids, lutein, zeaxanthin, vitamin C, vitamin E, and zinc are among the supplements examined for their potential eye health advantages.

However, supplements should be used with caution because they are not as strictly regulated as prescription drugs. Always contact with a healthcare expert before beginning any new supplement program, as they can help you determine the proper dosage and confirm that the supplements are safe and beneficial for your needs.

How Can I Stay Motivated and Consistent with My Diet Plan?

Maintaining motivation and consistency with a diet plan can be difficult, especially when confronted with temptation or difficulties. Here are some recommendations to keep you on track:

Set reasonable goals: Divide your nutritional goals into tiny, manageable steps. Celebrate your accomplishments along the road to keep motivated.

Find healthy substitutes: Rather than focusing on things to avoid, try new recipes and ingredients that fit your nutritional goals.

Plan ahead: Set aside time to plan and prepare your meals for the upcoming week.

Having healthy options readily available can assist in reducing impulsive meal decisions.

Stay accountable: Enlist the help of a friend, family member, or healthcare professional to keep you accountable and inspired.

Focus on the benefits: Remind yourself of how good food can improve your overall health and well-being, including your vision.

By implementing these tactics into your daily routine, you can improve your odds of staying motivated and consistent with your nutritional plan, so benefiting your eye health and general wellness.

CHAPTER SIX

Macular degeneration, which affects the center region of the retina (macula), has a substantial influence on eyesight and quality of life. While pharmacological interventions are critical, lifestyle changes play an important part in properly controlling the disease

This chapter focuses on providing persons with macular degeneration with practical ideas and tactics for maintaining their visual health in the long term.

The importance of regular eye exams and checkups

Regular eye exams are essential for people with macular degeneration. These checks allow for early diagnosis of any changes in vision or the course of the ailment. Monitoring the health of the macula and other regions of the eye allows eye care experts to intervene quickly, perhaps reducing or avoiding additional damage. In this part, we discuss the importance of scheduling and following to routine eye exams, allowing readers to take proactive steps to manage their eye health.

Protecting your eyes from harmful UV rays. UV radiation is a major hazard to eye health, worsening disorders such as macular degeneration. Individuals with this illness should incorporate UV protection measures into their daily lives. There are several ways to protect the eyes from damaging rays, including wearing sunglasses with UV-blocking lenses and wearing wide-brimmed hats. This section discusses the necessity of UV protection and provides practical recommendations for efficiently incorporating it into one's lifestyle.

Quitting Smoking: The Effect on Eye Health

Smoking is a well-known risk factor for macular degeneration, which can exacerbate its progression. Quitting smoking not only improves general health but also helps people with this condition maintain their vision. This section empowers readers by explaining the detrimental effects of smoking on eye health and providing information and help for quitting smoking.

Sleep Hygiene for Overall Wellness.

Quality sleep is critical for general well-being, including vision health. Poor sleep patterns can exacerbate pre-existing eye disorders, such as macular degeneration. This section discusses the importance of sleep hygiene habits such as sticking to a consistent sleep schedule, having a suitable sleep environment, and avoiding stimulants before bedtime. Individuals can improve their eye health and overall well-being by optimizing their sleep quality.

Incorporating Stress Relief Techniques into Daily Life

Chronic stress can harm eye health and exacerbate problems such as macular degeneration. As a result, incorporating stress-relief practices into one's daily routine is critical for effectively treating this illness. This section examines several stress-management practices, from mindfulness meditation to progressive muscle relaxation, and offers practical advice for incorporating them into daily routines. Individuals who reduce their stress levels can improve their eye health and general quality of life.

Finally, lifestyle changes are critical for managing long-term macular degeneration. By emphasizing the need for frequent eye exams, UV protection, smoking cessation, excellent sleep hygiene, and stress management, this chapter provides readers with the knowledge and skills they need to make proactive efforts to preserve their vision and optimize their overall well-being.

Reflecting on Your Trip So Far: As you near the end of the Glaucoma Prevention Diet Cookbook, take time to reflect on your trip thus far. Reflecting allows you to recognize your accomplishments, overcome obstacles, and identify areas for growth. Reflect on the dishes you've tried, the nutritional improvements you've made, and the lifestyle changes you've adopted. Take note of how these adjustments have impacted your entire well-being, including your eye health. Reflecting on your path provides significant information that can help you plan your future glaucoma prevention activities.

Setting Realistic Goals for Continuous Improvement: Reflection provides an opportunity to establish realistic goals for continuous improvement. Consider what you've learned about your food preferences, culinary habits, and lifestyle choices from this cookbook. Use this knowledge to set attainable goals that are consistent with your long-term vision for preventing glaucoma.

 Set clear, quantifiable, and reachable goals, whether they be to incorporate more leafy greens into your meals, reduce your sodium intake, or commit to regular exercise. Setting realistic goals prepares you for success and ensures that your efforts are focused and successful.

Celebrating Milestones and Achievements: As you attempt to avoid glaucoma through dietary and lifestyle changes, it's important to acknowledge and appreciate your progress.

Whether it's meeting a weight reduction goal, sticking to your new eating habits, or improving your general health, take the time to appreciate and celebrate your accomplishments. Celebrating milestones not only enhances morale and enthusiasm but also promotes great behavior. Share your accomplishments with friends and family, reward yourself for your efforts, and be proud of the progress you've made toward maintaining your eye health.

Adjusting Your Plan for Optimal Results: While the Glaucoma Prevention Diet Cookbook is a complete guide to dietary recommendations for avoiding glaucoma, it's important to remember that everyone's path is unique. As you progress towards ideal eye health, be prepared to change your approach as needed. Pay attention to how your body reacts to various foods, supplements, and lifestyle changes, and be prepared to adjust your strategy accordingly. If specific recipes or dietary advice don't work for you, don't be scared to look into other possibilities. Remember that flexibility is essential for long-term success, and be willing to alter your strategy to meet your specific needs and preferences.

Moving Forward with Confidence and Optimism: As you complete your journey with the Glaucoma Prevention Diet Cookbook, look ahead with confidence and optimism. With the knowledge, skills, and insights you've learned from this experience, you're ready to continue prioritizing your eye health and general well-being.

Approach each day with a positive attitude, understanding that each small move towards prevention is a step in the right direction. Stay committed to making healthy choices, stay up to date on the latest glaucoma research and advances, and take proactive steps to manage your eye health. With drive, perseverance, and a dose of optimism, you can empower yourself to live a healthy, glaucoma-free life.

Nourishing Meals and Snacks for Macular Degeneration Management

Salmon and Avocado Salad: A refreshing salad with salmon high in omega-3 fatty acids, avocado for healthy fats, and leafy greens for antioxidants like lutein and zeaxanthin.

Spinach and Berry Salad: A colorful salad made with spinach, berries (such as blueberries or raspberries), and nuts or seeds for extra crunch and nutrients. It contains vitamins, minerals, and antioxidants.

Vegetable and Lentil Soup: This hearty soup contains a range of vegetables such as carrots, tomatoes, and kale, as well as lentils for protein and fiber, which are necessary elements for eye health.

Quinoa & Roasted Vegetable dish: This nutritious dish contains quinoa, roasted veggies (such as bell peppers, sweet potatoes, and broccoli), and a drizzle of olive oil for healthy fats and antioxidants.

Baked Cod with Tomato and Olive Tapenade: In this Mediterranean-inspired recipe, cod provides lean protein and omega-3 fatty acids, while tomatoes and olives add antioxidants and flavor.

Egg & Vegetable Frittata: A flexible frittata made with eggs and a variety of colorful vegetables such as bell peppers, spinach, and mushrooms, which provide a variety of nutrients that are good for your eyes.

Chia Seed Pudding with Mixed Berries: A healthy and tasty dessert or snack cooked with chia seeds, almond milk, and mixed berries that contain omega-3 fatty acids, fiber, and antioxidants.

Turkey and Vegetable Stir-Fry: Lean turkey served with a variety of colorful vegetables stir-fried in a light sauce, providing protein, vitamins, minerals, and antioxidants in a delicious dish.

Broiled Asparagus with Lemon and Parmesan: Asparagus contains vitamins A, C, and E, as well as antioxidants like lutein and zeaxanthin. Broiling with lemon and Parmesan enhances flavor and nutrition.

Mango and Spinach Smoothie: A delightful smoothie with mango, spinach, Greek yogurt, and a splash of almond milk that contains vitamins, minerals, antioxidants, and probiotics.

30 Day to Healthy Vision: A Meal Plan for Managing Macular Degeneration with Delicious and Nutritious Meals"

Day 1:

Breakfast: Spinach and Berry Smoothie.

Snack: Carrot Sticks and Hummus.

Lunch: Vegetable and lentil soup.

Snack: Chia Seed Pudding with Mixed Berries.

Dinner: Salmon and avocado salad.

Day 2:

Breakfast: Egg and vegetable frittata.

Snack: Greek Yoghurt and Berries.

Lunch: Quinoa and roasted vegetable bowl.

Snack: Mango and spinach smoothie.

Dinner: Baked cod with tomato and olive tapenade.

Continue this pattern, ensuring that each day includes a variety of nutrient-rich foods, including fruits, vegetables, lean proteins, whole grains, and healthy fats. Adjust portion sizes based on individual calorie needs and preferences, and encourage hydration with water throughout the day. Patients should also consult with their healthcare provider or a registered dietitian for personalized dietary recommendations.

THE END